MEAL PREP FOR PREGNANT WOMEN

Nourishing your Pregnancy Journey

Roy Freeman

Table of Contents

Introduction

Hello from the realm of "Meal Prep for Pregnant Women"! Throughout the magical journey of pregnancy, this book is meant to be your trustworthy travel companion, providing precious insights into the critical connection between nutrition and the health of both you and your unborn child.

Pregnancy is a moment of life that brings with it a lot of physical and emotional changes, as well as anticipation and joy. Despite these changes, one thing has remained constant: the crucial importance of a balanced diet. When you are pregnant, your body is working very hard to support and foster the growth of a new life. Your diet has a big impact on both your health and the development of your unborn kid.

In this book, we delve thoroughly into the intricate network of pregnancy nutrition. We explore the intricate relationships between nutrients that support your growing body, promote healthy fetal development, and prepare you for the incredible journey that lies ahead. We stress the value of meal preparation because we understand that time is a scarce resource and that it may provide you with the comfort and confidence you need to manage the demands of pregnancy.

During pregnancy, one has to be more aware of nutritional needs. Every mouthful you eat lays the foundation for your baby's well-being. From the very first trimester to the absolute last second, your body needs a precise balance of vitamins, minerals, proteins, and other essential substances to support healthy development. We go through the specific nutrients that are crucial at various stages of pregnancy to assist you in making the best choices for both you and your unborn child.

You are aware of the time constraints and weariness that come with this particular stage of pregnancy. Here is where meal-planning magic comes into play. By spending a little time strategically planning your meals, you may enjoy a week's worth of good and balanced meals without having to deal with the hassle of regular cooking. We'll talk about the benefits and use of meal planning, particularly for expecting moms. Meal planning offers a wide range of advantages that may improve your health and the whole pregnancy process, from ensuring you have access to nutritional substitutes on hectic days to helping you curb cravings with thoughtful decisions.

As a result, whether you're a first-time parent navigating uncharted territory or a seasoned expert looking to enhance your pregnant journey, this book is here to assist you. Let's go on this adventure together armed with knowledge, compassion, and effective meal preparation techniques. One prepared meal at a time, be ready to experience a more fulfilling and healthier pregnancy.

Chapter

I

Essentials of Pregnancy Nutrition

As you begin this amazing journey of pregnancy, understanding the complexities of food becomes not just useful but crucial. This chapter will serve as your compass as you navigate the essential nutritional elements that provide the groundwork for a successful and healthy pregnancy.

Understanding Nutritional Needs During Pregnancy

During pregnancy, your body goes through several changes that all need certain nutrients to support the growth and development of your unborn child. We talk about the increased calorie and nutritional demands that come with each trimester, emphasizing the need to eat a balanced diet that satisfies both your needs and the needs of your growing child.

Important Nutrients for Mother and Baby discover the vital nutrients that maintain your well-being and encourage healthy fetal growth. So that you may make choices that are healthy for both you and your unborn child, we explain the functions of these nutrients and their sources in foods, covering everything from calcium and omega-3 fatty acids to folate and iron.

Suggested Daily Caloric Intake

Learn how your caloric needs change throughout pregnancy and how to strike the right balance to maintain a healthy weight increase. We give guidance on how to calculate your daily calorie intake based on your pre-pregnancy weight, amount of activity, and trimester to help you tailor your meal plan to match your requirements.

Managing Healthy Weight Gain

Although weight gain associated with pregnancy is unavoidable, it must be controlled to protect your health and the health of your unborn child. Learn the parameters for a healthy weight rise, how to maintain a healthy weight, and how a healthy diet relates to effective weight control.

In this chapter, we lay the groundwork for your journey into pregnant nutrition. Making better-educated choices that will feed both you and your growing kid may be made easier if you are aware of what your body needs in terms of nutrition. Understanding the food needs during pregnancy is the first step toward having a healthier and more rewarding pregnancy.

Adaptation to Changing Nutrient Demands

From the moment of conception, your body enters a dynamic state of growth and development. With each trimester, your nutritional requirements alter as well as those of your developing baby. We go into the tiny variances in dietary requirements to make sure you are educated on the precise vitamins, minerals, and macronutrients required for sustaining a healthy pregnancy.

The Best Fetal Development's Elements

Your baby's diet has a significant impact on how its organs, tissues, and overall health grow. The critical roles that nutrients like folic acid, iron, calcium, and protein play in promoting healthy embryonic development are examined in this article. Understanding how these dietary elements affect the health of your unborn kid will enable you to design a diet that nourishes the two of you.

Balance of Macronutrients for Energy and Wellness

Carbohydrates, proteins, and lipids, the three primary building blocks of a balanced diet, are significantly more important during pregnancy. To maintain your energy levels, manage weight gain, and ensure your baby's healthy development, learn how to balance these macronutrients.

What Micronutrients Do to Your Health

Even while vitamins and minerals are only needed in very small quantities, their significance cannot be overstated. We focus on the role of micronutrients in the immune system, bone health, brain development, and other processes. A few examples include zinc, omega-3 fatty acids, and vitamin D. You may pick a diet that is healthy for both you and your unborn child by understanding how these micronutrients influence your body.

Considering Special Dietary Considerations

When it comes to specific dietary considerations, including vegetarian or vegan diets, pregnancy calls for particular caution. To meet your increased nutritional needs and ensure that you and your baby get enough nourishment, we provide suggestions on how to adapt these meal selections.

The cornerstone of a healthy experience, as you navigate the pregnancy chapters, is having a solid understanding of your nutritional needs. Knowing the changing needs and the roles of various nutrients will help you make choices that will benefit both your health and the healthy development of your child.

Essential Vitamins for Mom and Baby

Your diet's nutrients play a big role in the intricate dance of pregnancy, promoting not just your health but also the growth and vitality of your developing kid. The crucial nutrients that provide the foundation for a successful and healthy pregnancy are highlighted in this chapter.

Folate Enhances Cellular Growth and Prevents Neural Tube Defects

Fast cell division and growth are made possible by the hero nutrition folate, often known as vitamin B9. We examine several folate-rich food sources to include in your diet for optimal maternal and fetal health and emphasize their importance in preventing neural tube defects in the first trimester.

Iron's Role in Increasing Blood and Oxygen Supply

Iron's importance during pregnancy is boosted because it encourages the production of red blood cells and ensures that oxygen is effectively delivered to both you and your unborn child. Learn how to cure iron deficiency anemia brought on by pregnancy and about easy-to-incorporate foods that are rich in iron.

Calcium Promotes Strong Bones and Heart Health

As your baby's bones and teeth grow, your calcium reserves are depleted. Learn how to maintain a balanced calcium intake to support these developments and to keep your bones and heart in excellent condition. We go through dietary calcium sources with you and show you how to appropriately prepare meals with them.

The Building Blocks of Life are Proteins

Protein takes center stage throughout pregnancy since it is essential for the growth of your unborn child's tissues and organs. Find out how to control your protein intake while adhering to a balanced diet, look into sources of high-quality protein, and be aware of your increased protein needs while pregnant.

Omega-3 Fatty Acids: Supporting Brain and Vision Development

The omega-3 fatty acid DHA in particular promotes your baby's brain and visual development. To promote your baby's cognitive and visual development, we examine the benefits of these essential fats, identify their sources, and provide suggestions on how to include them in your meals.

Iodine's Support for Thyroid Activity and Cognitive Growth

The production of thyroid hormones, which are necessary for both your metabolism and the development of your unborn child's brain, depends on iodine. Learn the value of iodine, how it contributes to a healthy pregnancy, and where to get iodine to add to your meal preparation routine.

Vitamin D improves Bone and Immune Health

Vitamin D supports calcium absorption and is crucial for a healthy immune system. We go through the importance of vitamin D during pregnancy, especially for the growth of your baby's bones, and provide suggestions on how to maintain optimum levels via dietary intake and sun exposure.

You'll be better able to create meal prep plans that are plentiful in the essential nutrients that support both you and your baby if you can identify the nutrients that are most important to your health. Instead of just being a period of growth, pregnancy offers a rare opportunity to intentionally choose one's food to nourish and nurture life.

Chapter

2

Beginning to prepare Meals

The best way to take care of your body throughout pregnancy and prepare for the challenges and benefits that lie ahead is via meal planning. In this chapter, the fundamentals of effective meal preparation are discussed, and you will leave with the abilities and information you need to apply this method to your journey of feeding both you and your growing kid.

The Rules of Meal Preparation

Welcome to meal preparation, a process that will alter the way you see nutrition throughout pregnancy. To help you navigate your pregnancy with comfort and nourishment, we delve into the basic concepts and techniques that serve as the foundation of effective meal planning in this chapter.

Discover the principles of food preparation and how it may transform your way of life. By using our detailed guidelines for planning, cooking, and storing meals beforehand, you can save the stress of last-minute meal planning and preparation.

Important Cooking Equipment

Learn about the tools and equipment in the kitchen that make food preparation fun, fast, and simple. We provide a comprehensive list of necessities, from storage containers to meal planning templates that will allow you to create an effective and well-organized meal prep area.

Making Meal Plans Using Trimesters

There are certain dietary restrictions and culinary considerations during pregnancy. We go through how to modify your meal planning to suit the varying requirements of each trimester. You'll be equipped to create food plans that complement your evolving journey, from overcoming morning sickness to supplying your body with more energy.

Picking Ingredients Carefully

Learn to shop with a purpose as you make decisions about the foods that will support your nutritional goals. Using fresh veggies, lean meats, whole grains, and other nutrient-dense foods as the foundation of your prepared meals is something we advise you to do.

Bringing together Flavors and Textures

Effective meal preparation requires variety in flavors and textures. Learn to balance the tastes and consistency of your prepared meals to keep your palate interested and content throughout the week.

Batch Cooking and Portion Control

Learn the art of batch cooking to produce larger quantities of food that may be consumed over several meals. To ensure that your meals have the right ratio of nutrients without being excessive, we also talk about portion control.

How to Tailor Your Diet to Your Cravings and Aversions

During pregnancy, a woman's food preferences and aversions often alter. Learn how to adjust your meal preparation to account for these variations so that your meals continue to be enjoyable and satisfying even as your appetites fluctuate.

You actively support your pregnancy self-care while also organizing your day by following the rules of effective food preparation. With a well-stocked kitchen, a strong plan, and a little creativity, you'll be well on your way to enjoying the benefits of meal preparation as you navigate this beautiful period of life.

Definition of Meal Preparation: A Time-Saving Method

As a time- and health-saving measure, learn the basics of food preparation. Meal planning, cooking, and portioning are covered in our discussion on meal preparation. You will always have healthy options accessible in this manner, regardless of how busy life becomes.

Selecting Recipes and Meals

Learn to choose recipes and meals that match your preferences and dietary requirements. We help you create a comprehensive and satisfying meal plan by directing you to balanced dishes that include crucial elements.

Your Step-by-Step Plan for Making a Meal

To establish a successful routine for meal preparation, master the art of meal planning. We go through how to organize your weekly menu to provide variety and a range of nutrients. From breakfast to snacks, we work with you to develop a plan that takes into account your shifting requirements throughout the trimester.

Purchasing Groceries Quickly

Prepare to make informed judgments before you go grocery shopping. We guide how to create a shopping list that matches your meal plan so that you can remain focused and organized while you browse the aisles.

Techniques for Freshness and Flavorful Preparation

Look into ways to cook meals that will keep them tasting good and being fresh. Even after your meals have been in the fridge for days, we provide tips on how to enhance their taste and quality. Marinating meats and blanching vegetables are examples of this.

Storage Techniques: Increasing Shelf Life [Discover the best storage practices to extend the shelf life of your cooked meals. We go through suitable containers, freezer guidelines, ingredient labeling, and rotation so you may reduce waste while maintaining the quality and enjoyment of your meals.

Manufacturing Productivity

Find out how assembly line cooking may speed up the preparation of your meals. We walk you through batch cooking and step-by-step preparation to demonstrate how to efficiently make several meals at once.

Schedules and Routines

Establishing a routine for meal preparation is the key to success. We provide suggestions on when to prepare meals so that they fit seamlessly into your schedule, whether it's a focused weekend session or a moderate everyday effort.

By mastering the essentials of food preparation, you're setting yourself up for a pregnancy marked by nourishment, convenience, and gourmet pleasure. The concepts you discover here will act as your guide as you start this phase of your life, allowing you to make the most of each meal for both you and your growing child.

Containers for Meal Preparation: Preserving Quality

Find out why it's crucial to choose the right containers for your prepared meals. We discuss the benefits of several container options, including glass and BPA-free plastic, as well as tips for portion control and lowering the risk of food contamination.

Cutting Tools: Precision and Efficiency

Find a selection of cutting tools to help you prepare food swiftly. We provide suggestions on how to ensure precision and safety when cooking meals, from using sharp knives to utilizing robust cutting boards.

Versatility of a Blender and Food Processor at Your Fingertips

Find out how blenders and food processors may make preparing meals simpler. We look at how these flexible appliances may help you create sauces, purees, and mixes, making them invaluable tools for creating nutrient-dense meals.

Use the Instant Pot and Slow Cooker to prepare food and then leave it alone

Learn more about the slow cookers and Instant Pots, which might be your companions in meal preparation. Learn how to use these tools effectively to produce tasty and healthful meals while reducing your workload and time commitment.

Tools for Measuring: Proportion Accuracy

To learn the skill of exact measurements, use a variety of measuring tools. We provide suggestions on how to ensure accurate portion sizes for your meals, promote a balanced diet, and utilize anything from measuring cups to kitchen scales.

Utilizing Flavors with Baking and Roasting Equipment

Learn about the benefits of baking and roasting for preparing meals as well as the necessary equipment. To give your prepared meals more variety and flavor, we go through oven-safe plates, baking sheets, and other items.

Options for Storage: Preserving Freshness

Discover innovative ways to store your food to keep it fresher and longer. We examine vacuum sealers, airtight packaging, and other tools that preserve the quality of your food by limiting exposure to air and moisture.

Templates for Meal Planning: Controlling Your Journey

To give your preparation process some structure, look into the realm of meal-planning templates and tools. We walk you through creating and executing your meal plans effectively utilizing printable templates, internet resources, and notebooks.

By assembling a collection of essential kitchen equipment and materials, you are empowering yourself to begin a road of efficient and productive food preparation. Similar to how a painter uses brushes and a canvas, these tools become your tools for producing delicious and healthful meals that support you and your unborn child during pregnancy.

Setting up Balanced Meals

It may be enjoyable and fulfilling to prepare meals that meet both your taste buds and the unique nutritional needs of pregnancy. To ensure that every bite supports a healthy and enjoyable pregnancy, this chapter dives into the art of preparing balanced meals that nourish both you and your growing child.

Ingredients in a Balanced Pregnancy Meal

Recognize the basic elements of a nutritious pregnancy meal. We look at how the fundamental nutrients—proteins, carbohydrates, healthy fats, vegetables, and fruits—affect both your overall health and the development of your unborn child.

Making Use of a Variety of Food Groups

Look into the benefits of having various nutrient-dense foods in your meals. Lean proteins, whole grains, dairy products or dairy alternatives, and colorful vegetables are just a few of the numerous nutritional categories that we guide you through while offering advice on how to prepare balanced and diverse meals.

Adjusting Your Diet for Each Trimester

Learn how to modify your meals' nutritional balance to suit the particular needs of each trimester. It's important to adjust your nutritional intake and quantities as your pregnancy progresses to ensure that your meals support both the development of your unborn child and your changing body.

Taking Care of Aversions and Cravings

Your dietary choices may change as a result of pregnancy-related changes in appetite and aversions. Learn coping skills for handling these changes, and tweak your meal planning to ensure you're still receiving a variety of nutrients even if your preferences shift.

Bringing together Flavors and Textures

As we explore the world of culinary harmony, learn how to blend flavors and textures in your meals. Learn how integrating sweet, savory, and umami tastes with a variety of textures can elevate your food preparation and make every bite a pleasurable and gratifying experience.

Calorie Balance and Portion Control with Awareness

Understand the importance of portion control while preparing balanced meals to promote a healthy weight increase during pregnancy. We guide determining portion sizes to ensure that your meals stick to your recommended calorie intake while still providing essential nutrients.

Hydration: An Underrated Hero

Consider the role that water plays in preparing a balanced diet. Since enough fluid consumption is essential for your health and the health of your unborn child, we provide advice on how to include hydrating beverages and meals rich in water into your meal preparation routine.

Making Meal Preparation Menus

Learn how to make everything work together by creating thorough meal preparation strategies. To help you navigate the challenges of creating balanced meals that meet your nutritional requirements, we provide sample menu options for each trimester.

As you create balanced meals, you are not only caring for your body and your unborn child; you are also encouraging a broader understanding of the enormous impacts that a healthy diet can have during pregnancy. By embracing the principles outlined in this chapter, you're laying the foundation for a healthy and happy culinary experience throughout your pregnancy.

Ingredients in a Balanced Pregnancy Meal

An important act of self-care during pregnancy is preparing meals that will nourish both you and your unborn child. This chapter will deconstruct the basic components of a balanced pregnancy meal to assist you in ensuring that each dish you prepare is a harmonious combination of essential nutrients, flavors, and textures.

Proteins are the Building Blocks of Growth

Embrace the significance of including high-quality proteins in your meals. Proteins support your body's needs during this time of change and aid in the development of your unborn child's tissues. We examine lean protein sources including chicken, fish, lentils, and tofu, and provide suggestions for cooking with them.

Utilizing Carbohydrates to Maintain Energy Levels

Consider how carbohydrates could be the primary source of energy for both your body and your growing child. We investigate the gradual energy release and fiber content of complex carbohydrates, which are present in whole grains, fruits, and vegetables and may aid in blood sugar regulation.

Good Fats are Nutrient Powerhouses

Learn the benefits of having healthy fats in your diet while pregnant. These fats increase meal absorption, support your baby's brain growth, and provide you with long-lasting pleasure. We go through the benefits of sources including avocados, almonds, seeds, and olive oil, as well as how to include them in your diet.

Nutrient-Rich Delights: Fruits and Vegetables

Learn about the colorful world of fruits and vegetables, which are all brimming with antioxidants, vitamins, and minerals that promote overall well-being. We discuss the benefits of various produce options and provide creative ways to make meals with them to increase their nutritional worth.

Nutrient Powerhouses: Good Fats

Find out why having healthy fats in your diet during pregnancy is beneficial. These fats promote nutrition absorption, aid in the development of your baby's brain, and provide you with long-lasting pleasure. We discuss how to include foods like olive oil, seeds, avocados, and almonds into your diet.

Delicious Nutrient-Rich Fruits and Vegetables

Discover the vibrant world of fruits and vegetables, which are loaded with nutrients that support general health, such as antioxidants, vitamins, and minerals. We go through the advantages of different crop selections and provide inventive recipes to use to generate more nutrient-dense meals.

Vital for Health is Water

Consider the value of water as a crucial component of a healthy pregnant diet. We discuss the need to be hydrated all day long and examine foods rich in water content, such as fruits, and vegetables.

Getting the Right Portion Size Balance

Learn the art of adjusting portion sizes to make sure your meals during pregnancy match your nutritional needs. We provide tips on selecting the proper portion sizes for each component of a balanced meal to encourage caloric balance and optimal nutrient intake.

You may make meals that will save your hunger while also advancing the growth of your unborn kid and your overall health if you know the purpose of each component in a balanced pregnancy meal. Embrace the beauty of combining proteins, carbohydrates, healthy fats, vegetables, fruits, fiber, and water to make meals that are tasty and satisfying.

Chapter

3

Pregnancy Recipes for Meal Prep

We cordially welcome you to our collection of meal prep recipes where you will find support for your health and the growth of your unborn child. We provide you with a broad range of flavors, textures, and nutrients to relish in recipes that have been thoughtfully created to satisfy the unique nutritional needs of each trimester in this chapter.

Feeding the First Trimester's Early Stages

Learn about recipes that have been selected with the demands and appetites of the first trimester in mind. We provide nourishing meals that are easy on the stomach, alleviate morning sickness, and ensure you get the essential nutrients you and your developing baby need at this critical time.

How to Stay Active in the Second Trimester

Find meals that satisfy the second trimester's increasing energy needs. These meals are designed to provide you with sustained energy as you reach the middle of your pregnancy, support your baby's rapid growth, and feed your growing body.

In the Third Trimester, Getting Ready for the Home Stretch

In the third trimester, as you prepare to give birth and greet your baby, look for recipes to aid you. The nutritious value of these meals is stressed, and they also promote healthy weight growth and include ingredients that ease common aches and pains.

Our recipes provide for the various dietary requirements that each trimester presents. We carefully considered the changing needs of both you and your child while creating our recipes, which vary from protein-rich meals to fiber-rich dishes and nutrient-dense snacks.

Selecting the Proper Macronutrients for Each Meal

Master the art of balancing the major nutrients in each meal. To ensure that every meal offers a balanced mix of nutrients that promote general well-being, we discuss the purposeful inclusion of proteins, carbohydrates, and healthy fats.

Utilizing Colorful Produce

Discover the benefits of using a range of colorful fruits and vegetables in your meals. We look at the nutrients present in different colors and talk about creative ways to add them to your meals for taste and visual appeal.

Consuming Filling Snacks between Meals

Find a variety of wholesome and substantial snacks that provide the perfect intermission between your main meals. We emphasize nutrient-dense foods that keep you energized and full all day.

Drinks that Make You More Hydrated

Find suggestions for revitalizing and hydrating beverages to enhance your fluid intake. To boost your general health, we offer enticing and beneficial alternatives to ordinary water, such as herbal teas and infused waters.

By using these meal prep recipes, you may enhance each day of your pregnancy with flavor, nutrition, and care. These dishes are more than just recipes; they're a celebration of your commitment to feeding yourself and your kid healthfully, one bite at a time.

Feeding the First Trimester's Early Stages

Congratulations on starting your incredible pregnancy journey! The first trimester is a time of immense growth and transformation as you begin to care for the valuable life growing inside of you. In this chapter, we provide a selection of meal prep recipes designed to fit the unique needs and challenges of the first trimester, ensuring that you are well-fed and supported throughout this crucial early time.

Nutritional Knowledge for the First Trimester

As you embark on this journey, you must be aware of the food needs during the first trimester. We discuss the significance of nutrients that are crucial for boosting your baby's rapid neural tube development and growth, such as folate, iron, and B vitamins.

Food Therapy for Morning Sickness

Early on in pregnancy, nausea and morning sickness are rather typical. We provide meals that place a light emphasis on nutrition so that it doesn't overwhelm your senses. These meals have flavors and nutrients that are simple to digest, which might lessen discomfort.

Getting to Energy Balance

As your body adjusts to the changes of pregnancy, weariness is a regular companion in the first trimester. Our meals are designed to provide you with steady energy from complex carbohydrates and lean proteins so that you can fend off exhaustion and maintain your vigor.

Recipes for First Trimester Meal Preparation

Creamy oatmeal with berries is a warm and satisfying breakfast option that is high in fiber, iron, and antioxidants to get your day started.

Gingered Carrot and Sweet Potato Soup is a soothing, nutrient-rich soup that also has the added benefit of easing motion sickness.

Chickpea and Quinoa Salad: a salad that is high in protein, has a lot of vegetables and herbs and provides delicious crunch and valuable nutrients.

Baked salmon with roasted vegetables is a wholesome dinner option that gives the vegetables a variety of vitamins and omega-3 fatty acids for brain growth.

Consuming Hydrating Food and Drinks

We also emphasize the need to stay hydrated throughout this trimester and provide suggestions for hydrating foods and beverages to maintain optimal fluid balance.

By using the recipes in this chapter to nourish your body, you may enter parenting with care and purpose. These meals not only provide you with the nutrients you need but also a sense of stability and comfort, helping you to confront the stunning but challenging terrain of the first trimester with vitality and nourishment.

Accepting the increase in Energy Requirements

During the second trimester, your baby undergoes substantial growth and development, increasing the amount of energy needed. We discuss the importance of feeding your body a variety of nutrients to keep your energy levels up and provide your child with the building blocks they need to thrive.

Important Nutrients of the Second Trimester

Look at the nutrients that are crucial right now. We delve into the significance of various minerals, from iron to calcium and omega-3 fatty acids, in maintaining both your health and your baby's ongoing growth.

Recipes for Meal Prep in the Second Trimester, as Examples

The spinach and berry smoothie is a wholesome morning pick-me-up that blends the advantages of leafy greens with antioxidant-rich berries for a vivacious start to your day.

A grilled chicken and quinoa bowl is a wholesome lunch option that offers lean protein, complex carbohydrates, and a variety of colorful greens for essential vitamins and minerals.

Salad with salmon and avocado: A nutritious, full, and light dinner salad with a mix of greens and vegetables, omega-3 fatty acids, and good fats.

Greek yogurt parfaits combine Greek yogurt with fruit, nuts, and other nutritious ingredients to provide sustained energy. They are a tasty, protein-rich snack.

A delicious and nutrient-dense dinner option, sweet potato and black bean tacos will provide you and your kid with fiber, vitamins, and plant-based proteins.

Support for Digestive Health

As your kid grows, your digestive system experiences more stress. We provide meals that include fiber-rich ingredients to encourage healthy digestion and lessen some of the common discomforts felt during this trimester.

Drinks High in Nutrients and Water

Learn about hydrating, nutrient-rich drinks that mix well with meals and help you stay properly hydrated, which is important for maintaining your energy levels.

By nourishing yourself with the dishes in this chapter, you may approach the second trimester with the vitality and strength you need to thrive. In addition to providing the essential nutrition your body and the growing baby need, these meals offer you a sense of fullness and confidence as you navigate this magnificent period of pregnancy.

In the Third Trimester, Getting Ready for the Home Stretch

As you approach the end of your pregnancy, your body is working hard to prepare for the delivery of your child. There are particular dietary considerations and needs during the third trimester. This chapter includes several meal prep recipes that are meant to help you throughout the third trimester. The meals stress healthy weight growth, nutritional density, and preparing you for childbirth and motherhood.

Taking Care of Nutritional Needs

During the third trimester, while your body is preparing for labor and delivery, your baby's development is at its quickest. At this point, we discuss the specific dietary requirements, emphasizing the importance of minerals like calcium, protein, and fiber.

How to Put On Healthy Weight While Keeping Your Energy Up

As your baby gains weight, maintaining a healthy weight increase becomes increasingly crucial. We discuss how eating a balanced diet may assist you in achieving this goal and provide examples of meals that have a combination of complex carbohydrates, proteins, and good fats to provide you with sustained energy.

Enhancing Comfort and Minimizing Discomfort

The third trimester is often accompanied by bodily discomforts such as heartburn, back pain, and swelling. You'll discover ingredients in our recipes that may help with pain alleviation as well as nutrients for your overall health.

Meal Preparation examples during the third Trimester

A comforting, hearty breakfast option that is packed with fiber, protein, and other essential nutrients is baked oatmeal with nuts and dried fruit. You'll have a good start on the day.

A full, healthy, and well-balanced lunch option that is high in vitamins, minerals, and plant-based protein is roasted vegetable and chickpea salad.

Vegetable and lentil stew is a hearty dish full of fiber, protein, and a variety of vegetables to help with digestion.

Nut butter and banana energy bites are a snack that gives you quick energy, healthy fats, and essential nutrients to keep you active between meals.

In the last few weeks of your pregnancy, consider soothing herbal infusions to help you unwind, relax, and promote a sense of tranquility.

Preparing for Childbirth and Beyond

We provide meals that give your body the vital nutrition it needs to maintain health and strength as you prepare for birth and the change from woman to mother.

Foods that Hydrate and Water

Find suggestions for hydrating meals and beverages as your pregnancy draws to a close to help you avoid fluid retention and maintain the proper amount of hydration.

The rapid energy, healthy fats, and vital nutrients in nut butter and banana energy bits will keep you active between meals.

Consider calming herbal infusions in the latter weeks of your pregnancy to help you relax, unwind, and encourage a feeling of tranquility.

Getting Ready for Birth and Beyond

As you get ready for labor and the transition from woman to mother, we serve meals that provide your body with the essential nourishment it needs to maintain health and vigor.

Water and Hydrating Foods

As your pregnancy comes to an end, find ideas for hydrating foods and drinks to help you minimize fluid retention and maintain the right level of hydration.

Preventing Typical Pregnancy Symptoms by Staying Hydrated

Hydration may be a powerful tool for managing some of the pregnancy's symptoms, which often come with their fair share of discomforts. We examine how being hydrated may help during morning sickness, prevent UT infections, and ease constipation.

Impact on the Baby's Development

Find out how your level of hydration affects your child's development directly. By exploring how adequate fluid intake supports placental function, nutrient transfer, and general fetal growth, we investigate the critical role that water plays in supporting a successful pregnancy.

Modifications and Hydration Requirements

When you get pregnant, your body requires different amounts of liquid. We guide how to identify your specific hydration needs during pregnancy and how to adjust these needs as you go through the several trimesters.

Symptoms of Dehydration

Recognizing the signs of dehydration is the first step in proactive self-care. We discuss common dehydration symptoms and guide how to determine when your body needs more water.

Things to Eat and Drink to Rehydrate

To aid in your efforts to maintain proper hydration, look into a variety of hydrating foods and beverages. We provide substitutes that make drinking water enjoyable and delectable, such as water-rich fruits and vegetables, herbal teas, and infused beverages.

Strategies for Keeping Hydrated

By adding practical strategies to your daily routine, you may learn how to maintain optimal hydration. We provide tips on how to set reminders, carry a reusable water bottle, and flavor your water to make staying hydrated an easy and enjoyable part of your day.

Water Consumption While Preparing Food

Look at the connection between meal preparation and hydration. We provide suggestions on how to include hydrating foods and beverages into your pre-made meals so that your hydration and nutritional goals are met.

By embracing the knowledge of hydration, you are giving your body and your unborn child the gift of nourishment. With the information and resources in this chapter, you can make being hydrated an important part of your pregnancy journey and meet your body's requirements for health, vitality, and well-being.

Making Healthy Drinks that Will Hydrate You

It's crucial to keep in mind that satisfying your thirst allows you to provide your body nourishment it needs. We go into the topic of hydrating and nourishing beverages in this chapter and provide you with a variety of recipes that will not only help you stay hydrated but will also benefit your pregnancy with a mouthwatering array of benefits.

The Effects of Drinks That Rehydrate

Learn about the mysterious realm of hydration and how it may rejuvenate your body. We discuss the importance of fluids for maintaining overall health, aiding in digestion, and promoting the smooth working of bodily systems.

Keeping Hydrated Away from Water

The finest hydrator is water, although a broad range of other beverages may help you keep hydrated. We investigate a range of options, each with a unique set of benefits, from herbal teas and flavored drinks to healthy smoothies.

Suitable Smoothies for Pregnancy

Learn about the advantages of smoothies as a hydrating and nutrient-rich option during pregnancy. We provide a variety of smoothie recipes that combine fruits, vegetables, proteins, and healthy fats to create delectable combinations that satisfy your specific needs for each trimester.

Flavorful Waters that Are Refreshing

Learn the art of adding flavors from the bounty of nature to water. We provide unique fruit, herb, and even vegetable combinations that improve the taste of water and make it more delightful to drink.

Herbal Teas for Relaxation and Wellness

Learn about herbal tea's relaxing properties and how they may help you relax while alleviating common pregnancy discomforts. The benefits of chamomile, ginger, peppermint, and other herbal beverages used to support your health are discussed.

Hydrating Snacks are Foods with High Water Content

Look into foods that are high in water so they can complement your hydration beverages. We look at meals that are hydrating, such as yogurt-based snacks and fruits like watermelon and cucumber.

Including Drinks in the Making of Meals

Learn how to include hydration drinks in the process of preparing meals. We include directions for preparing large volumes of infused waters, herbal teas, and smoothie ingredients to make it easier for you to stay hydrated.

Conscious Drinking for Wellness

Learn to carefully hydrate by paying attention to your body's signals and giving it water as needed. For your optimum well-being, we provide suggestions on how to integrate this knowledge into your daily activities.

Using the recipes and methods in this chapter, you may turn to keep hydrated into an enjoyable and healthy habit. These beverages satisfy your thirst while also enhancing your pregnancy with a symphony of tastes, benefits, and aromas. You and your kid experience vitality, well-being, and tenderness after consuming these mixtures that extend beyond simple drunkenness.

Preparing Meals during Pregnancy

Greetings on the arrival of your beloved kid! As you go into the postpartum period, it's more important than ever to nourish your body. We delve into the topic of postpartum meal planning in this transformative chapter, offering you suggestions and recipes to support your recovery, nursing experience, and overall well-being.

Postpartum Nutrition for Women: A Crucial Aspect

Understanding the unique nutritional needs of the postpartum period is crucial for promoting breastfeeding and assisting your body's recovery following birth. We discuss the nutrients that are crucial for healing, maintaining energy, and promoting a consistent milk supply for your infant.

Maintaining a Balance between Nutrition and Recovery

Examine how to strike a balance between self-care and nutrition throughout the postpartum period. We provide suggestions on how to prioritize your needs while ensuring that you are strong and well-nourished enough to care for your kid.

Promoting Lactation and Breastfeeding

If you are nursing, the health of your infant and your nutritional needs are tightly tied. We go through foods that are known to promote lactation when you start your breastfeeding journey and offer recipes that employ these ingredients.

Examples of Postpartum Meal Prep Recipes

Since it is packed with vegetables, lean protein, and nourishing broth, Hearty Vegetable, and Chicken Soup is a calming, nutrient-dense soup that is ideal for postpartum recovery.

Flaxseed and oatmeal breakfast bowl: Your postpartum needs for sustained energy, fiber, and essential nutrients will be satisfied by this meal.

Salad with salmon and spinach: A wholesome lunch option that contains the vitamins, iron, and omega-3 fatty acids found in leafy greens.

The quinoa and chickpea power bowl is a nutrient-dense lunch option that offers protein, complex carbohydrates, and several other essential elements for your recovery.

The lactation smoothie, which contains oats, flaxseeds, and berries among other nutritious and delicious ingredients, is meant to promote breastfeeding.

Self-care and Water Intake

Examine the role that water plays in your recovery and nursing experience throughout the postpartum period. We talk about the importance of being hydrated and provide suggestions for hydrating meals and beverages.

Balanced Nutrition and Convenience

Learn how to blend convenience and nutrition during the demanding postpartum period. We discuss the benefits of using meal planning templates, keeping wholesome snacks on hand, and cooking meals that can be frozen to make your postpartum diet simpler.

By implementing the postpartum meal planning recommendations and recipes in this chapter, you are giving yourself the gift of nourishment, recovery, and well-being. These meals support not only your physical recovery but also your emotional well-being as you embark on the beautiful journey of parenthood. As you take care of your baby, remember that feeding yourself is a nice act that benefits you and your kid.

Chapter

4

Permanent Healthy Eating Patterns

Congratulations! You are now entering a new era when diet is still very essential, after passing through the stages of pregnancy and postpartum. The development of lifelong, healthy eating habits that will benefit you and your family for many years is the topic of this chapter. These behaviors need to be enduring throughout life stages.

Accepting Nutrition for Life

Learn how crucial it is to switch from short-term goals to long-term, sustainable healthy eating routines. We discuss the transformative power of seeing nutrition as a lifelong journey rather than a one-time activity.

Building a Solid Foundation

Discover how to keep a balanced diet. We talk about the importance of eating a variety of nutrient-dense meals, being mindful of how much you eat, and sometimes indulging in pleasures while keeping an eye on your overall health.

Mindful Eating for Connection

Learn about mindful eating and how it could help you develop a stronger connection with your food, your body, and your overall well-being. We provide suggestions on how to savor each bite, recognize symptoms of hunger and fullness, and make mealtimes special.

Family-Centered Nutrition

Your loved ones will need to adopt a healthy food routine as your family grows. We discuss strategies to include your family in meal preparation, from introducing new foods to developing a healthy eating routine.

Making Meal Planning and Preparation a Habit

Consider the possibility that the skills you have acquired in food preparation and planning throughout pregnancy and beyond may become lifelong habits. We guide how to maintain meal planning, adapt recipes to fit various needs, and keep your kitchen tidy.

Understanding Your Body's Wisdom

Learn to eat intuitively, which encourages you to pay attention to your body's cues and choose meals that suit your particular needs and preferences. We teach you how to recognize and honor your body's indications.

Maintaining Hydration and Being Healthy

Hydration is still crucial for optimum health even throughout pregnancy and the postpartum period. We discuss how to maintain your habits for drinking water and consider the long-term benefits of doing so.

Taking Life and Food Easily

Discover the joy of enjoying both food and life. We discuss the connection between good nutrition and gratitude as well as the importance of embracing cultural diversity in food and eating customs.

By establishing lifelong healthy eating habits, you are embarking on a lifetime journey of self-care, vitality, and well-being. These actions show how committed you are to caring for your family and yourself, as well as how well your diet and way of life complement one another. As you develop these habits, you are not only preserving your physical health but also leaving behind a legacy of well-being that extends well beyond the confines of this book.

Maintaining Nutritional Decisions after Giving Birth

Congratulations on completing the incredible adventure of pregnancy and motherhood! When you transition to postpartum life, your commitment to your health and well-being will still be evident. We'll look at how to maintain and integrate your pregnancy-related food habits into your routine in this chapter.

Accepting Stability

In your search for a healthy diet, learn to be consistent. We discuss how your newly established healthy eating habits may support your well-being and vitality for the rest of your life.

Putting Self-Care First

When your life changes, it's essential to continue prioritizing your own needs. We look at the relationship between nourishing your body correctly and taking care of your physical, emotional, and mental well-being.

Getting Experience in New Roles

When your kid is born, your parental obligation becomes more important. We discuss how to look after your family and maintain a healthy diet. We also provide advice on how to prepare meals that the entire family will like as well as creative ways to include healthful foods into your everyday routine.

Keeping Your Stamina and Energy

Maintaining your energy and endurance is crucial because of the potential demands of postpartum life. We look at how nutrient-dense foods, well-balanced meals, and the right amount of water affect your energy and stamina.

Making Mindful Choices during Change

The time after childbirth ushers in new routines, challenges, and joys. We discuss mindful eating and how it could enable you to make conscientious food choices despite life's ups and downs.

Investigating Food's New Horizons

As you continue your culinary voyage, discover new ingredients, cuisines, and experiences. We discuss the benefits of eating a variety of meals and how doing so might enhance your nutritional experience.

Managing Food and Indulgence

Learn the art of balance as you continue on your nutritious journey. We discuss strategies for indulging in pleasures while establishing a foundation of foods high in nutrients.

Taking Good Care of Your Health Now and in the Future

Your long-term health is an investment, so keep up your food choices. We go through the long-term health benefits and discuss how maintaining a commitment to good eating improves your overall quality of life.

As you transition from pregnancy to postpartum life, your strategy for self-care and nourishment alters. By using the information in this chapter, you're helping to build a foundation for your family's long-term health and pleasure. Every meal you eat and every choice you make becomes a thread in the continuous story of your life—a story of energy, nutrition, and a commitment to seeing health as a lifelong adventure.

Setting Positive Example for Your Child

Parenting is much more than just providing for your child's needs. Your choices, particularly those related to eating, have a big influence on how they see their health and well-being. In this chapter, we look at the many advantages of teaching your kids good food and nutrition practices.

Setting a High Standard

Learn how your actions impact your child's attitudes and eating habits. We highlight the importance of setting an example for mindful eating and good food choices by explaining how youngsters often mimic the habits they witness in adults.

How to Establish a Healthy Relationship with Food

Learn why it's crucial to provide your child with a favorable relationship with food at an early age. We discuss how the way you see food, body image, and self-care may have a significant effect on how your children perceive these issues.

What Is Diversity in Nutrients?

Discover the advantages of introducing your child to a range of foods at a young age. We discuss how exposing children to a range of flavors, textures, and foods may foster in them a more open-minded palate and a better understanding of nutrition.

Developing a Love of Cooking

Consider the benefits of having your child assist you in the kitchen. We discuss how preparing healthy meals may encourage a sense of responsibility, creativity, and pride.

Navigating Picky Eating Patiently

For many children, picky eating tends to come in waves, which may be challenging for parents. We provide advice on how to handle picky eating with patience, understanding, and strategies that encourage healthy eating habits.

Fostering Positive Body Image

Talk to your child about the value of promoting a positive body image. We examine techniques for teaching young people to respect their bodies and the importance of focusing on one's health and well-being rather than external attractiveness.

Collaboration and Open Discussion

Discuss honestly with your child food, nutrition, and general health. We guide how to respond to inquiries, dispel myths, and promote an environment where learning about nutrition is a shared experience.

By setting a good example for them with your eating practices, you may teach your child valuable lessons that extend well beyond the dinner table. The choices you make, the attitudes you display, and the values you instill will form your child's connection with food, health, and self-care. As you guide them on this journey, you are doing more than simply providing for their physical needs; you are also developing their capacity to lead balanced, considerate, and healthy lives.

Conclusion

As the last chapter of the book approaches, you've been on a wonderful journey of nurturing both you and your growing kid through the life-changing phases of pregnancy, postpartum, and beyond. Because of your commitment to your health, well-being, and the art of meal preparation, every bite you've prepared and treasured has been woven into a tapestry of care, purpose, and love.

Let's think about what you took away from this book, what you experienced, and what you realized and learned in this last chapter:

You give yourself and your kid nutrition as a gift, as a tangible expression of self-love and care. It does more than just provide your body energy. Every meal, snack, and sip of water is an opportunity to give your body and mind a burst of vitality.

By engaging in mindful eating, which has taught you to savor each bite and pay attention to your body's signals, you have cultivated a deeper connection with your food. Your health will benefit from this activity, and eating will also be more pleasant.

Even on the busiest of days, you can properly nourish your body because you've perfected the art of meal preparation. You've set up comfort, health, and balance by planning, organizing, and preparing your meals.

The settings of pregnancy, postpartum, and other phases have changed as you move through them. Your ability to adapt your nutritional preferences to suit the unique needs of each phase demonstrates your resiliency, adaptability, and commitment to self-care.

As you go from one level to another, the habits you've established follow you. These habits—from being adequately hydrated to balancing your macronutrient intake—continue to point you in the direction of your best health and well-being.

By establishing a good example for yourself and your family, you're nurturing a legacy of good health that will last for decades. Your choices now will determine a future filled with health, vitality, and conscientious living.

As you finish this chapter and go on into the world, may you carry with you the wisdom, abilities, and nourishment you have gained. Your journey toward self-care and mindful eating is ongoing, and you should use every opportunity to travel it. Remember that every meal is an opportunity to nourish not just your physical needs but also your spirit, general well-being, and aspirations for a life filled with strength and joy.

Thank you for packing this book for your vacation. As you continue to take care of yourself and your family, may the nutritious route ahead offer you courage, joy, and a deep sense of fulfillment.

Appendix

Rules for Shopping Lists

Making a well-organized shopping list is one of the most crucial processes in completing meal preparation and ensuring that you have the supplies on hand to support your nutritional goals. By using this advice, you can streamline your shopping, maximize your time and resources, and guarantee that your kitchen is fully stocked with everything you need for a healthy week.

Examine your weekly menu: Review your weekly menu before creating a shopping list. List the ingredients you'll need for each meal, including the main dish, sides, snacks, and beverages.

Organize Items by Category: Your shopping list should be divided into categories such as fruits, vegetables, proteins, dairy, grains, pantry basics, and snacks. You'll find it simpler to do business and can be sure you won't miss anything crucial if you do this.

Check Having a Pantry Before you go shopping, check your pantry, fridge, and freezer to see what you already have. This reduces food waste and eliminates repetitive actions.

Think on nutrient diversity on your shopping list, be sure to include a variety of nutrient-dense foods. Choose a variety of fresh fruits and vegetables, nutritious grains, lean proteins, good fats, dairy items, and dairy replacements.

Consider Portion Proportions: Consider portion proportions while adding items to your list. For instance, if a recipe calls for a specific quantity of quinoa, be sure to get the appropriate quantity to prevent overspending on the ingredient.

Remember to Drink: Water intake should be maintained. Include beverages that will keep you hydrated, such as water, herbal teas, and fruit for water infusions or smoothie ingredients.

Examine your recipes to determine if any unique or special ingredients are required. Don't forget to include them in your shopping list to avoid hurried trips to the store.

Consider Food Storage: If you wish to prepare food ahead of time-for example, by chopping vegetables or portioning meat-consider food storage needs. Be sure to include any necessary containers or bags on your list.

Examine the Expiry Dates: When possible, choose items with a longer shelf life, but keep expiry dates in mind as well. Buy perishables sparingly and in small quantities.

Make a shopping list: Follow your shopping list while you are at the store. Avoid making impulsive purchases that conflict with your dietary and health goals.

As necessary, adjust: Be prepared to change your list if you find alternatives or substitutions while shopping. If you are adaptable, you could benefit from amazing deals or fresh food.